Psoriasis Diet Guide

The Role of Diet in Managing Psoriasis

By

Cedric Dairmid

Table of Contents

CHAPTER 1
Introduction

1.1 Understanding Psoriasis

Psoriasis is a chronic skin condition that affects millions of people worldwide. It is characterized by the rapid growth of skin cells, leading to the formation of red, scaly, and often itchy patches on the skin. These patches can appear anywhere on the body, but they are most commonly found on the elbows, knees, scalp, and lower back. While the visible symptoms of psoriasis manifest on the skin, it is essential to recognize that psoriasis is not merely a skin issue. It is, in fact, an autoimmune condition with a complex and multifaceted nature.

Psoriasis results from an overactive immune response. In a healthy immune system, white blood cells are responsible for defending the body against foreign invaders such as bacteria and viruses. However, in people with psoriasis, these immune cells mistakenly attack healthy skin cells. This attack triggers a series of events, including inflammation, an accelerated skin cell production cycle, and the characteristic scaling and redness associated with the condition. The exact cause of psoriasis is still not fully understood, but genetics, environmental factors, and the immune system all play a role in its development.

One of the defining features of psoriasis is its unpredictable and chronic nature. People living with psoriasis often experience flare-ups, periods when their symptoms worsen, followed by periods of remission where symptoms subside or improve. The severity of psoriasis can vary widely from person to person, with some individuals experiencing mild, localized patches, while others may have extensive involvement that affects their overall quality of life.

Psoriasis is not merely a cosmetic concern; it can have a significant impact on a person's physical and emotional well-being. The visible nature of the condition can lead to self-esteem issues, social stigma, and psychological distress. Many individuals with psoriasis experience feelings of self-consciousness and embarrassment, which can further exacerbate the stress associated with the condition.

In addition to the skin, psoriasis can also affect other areas of the body, including the joints. Psoriatic arthritis is a related condition where inflammation and joint pain occur alongside skin symptoms. The management of psoriasis often requires a holistic approach that considers both the skin and joint aspects of the condition.

Understanding the complexity of psoriasis is the first step in effectively managing it. While there is no cure for psoriasis, various treatment options are available to control symptoms, reduce inflammation, and promote healing. Medications, phototherapy, and lifestyle modifications are common strategies employed by healthcare professionals to help individuals manage their psoriasis effectively.

1.2 The Role of Diet in Managing Psoriasis

Diet plays a vital role in the management of psoriasis. While psoriasis is primarily an autoimmune condition, the foods we consume can influence the inflammatory response in our bodies, potentially triggering or exacerbating symptoms. It's important to note that there is no one-size-fits-all diet for psoriasis because the condition varies from person to person. However, research and clinical experiences suggest that dietary choices can impact the severity of psoriasis and the frequency of flare-ups.

The relationship between diet and psoriasis is intrinsically linked to inflammation. Inflammation is the body's natural response to injury or infection, but chronic inflammation is often associated with autoimmune conditions like psoriasis. Certain foods can promote inflammation, while others have anti-inflammatory properties. For individuals with psoriasis, the goal is to minimize pro-inflammatory foods and incorporate anti-inflammatory choices into their diet.

Pro-inflammatory foods to be cautious of include processed foods high in sugar and unhealthy fats, red meat, and dairy products. Excessive alcohol consumption and smoking can also worsen inflammation. On the other hand, anti-inflammatory foods include fruits and vegetables rich in antioxidants, whole grains, lean proteins, and sources of healthy fats like nuts, seeds, and fatty fish.

Omega-3 fatty acids, found in fish such as salmon, mackerel, and sardines, have received particular attention for their potential benefits in managing psoriasis. These fatty acids have anti-inflammatory properties and may help reduce the severity of symptoms. Furthermore, vitamins and minerals, especially vitamin D, vitamin A, and zinc, are essential for skin health and can play a role in managing psoriasis symptoms.

Hydration is another critical aspect of dietary management for psoriasis. Proper hydration ensures that the skin remains moist and can help prevent dryness and itching, common complaints among those with psoriasis. Drinking an adequate amount of water is essential, and including water-rich foods like cucumbers and watermelon in your diet can also contribute to hydration.

The link between diet and psoriasis is undeniable, and it offers individuals with psoriasis an opportunity to take an active role in managing their condition. While dietary changes alone may not be a cure for psoriasis, they can complement other treatment strategies and potentially lead to more manageable symptoms and improved quality of life. This guide aims to explore the intricacies of the psoriasis-diet connection, providing information, tips, and strategies to help individuals make informed dietary choices that support their journey toward healthier skin and well-being.

CHAPTER 2

Psoriasis and Nutrition

2.1 How Nutrition Impacts Psoriasis

Understanding how nutrition impacts psoriasis is crucial for individuals living with this chronic skin condition. While psoriasis is fundamentally an autoimmune disorder, the foods we consume can have a significant influence on the development and severity of symptoms. The relationship between nutrition and psoriasis revolves around the role of inflammation, the immune system, and the maintenance of healthy skin.

- **Inflammation**: Psoriasis is characterized by chronic inflammation. The immune system's response is overactive, causing an ongoing cycle of inflammation and skin cell turnover. Nutrition plays a pivotal role in modulating this inflammatory response. Certain foods, particularly those high in sugar, unhealthy fats, and processed ingredients, can exacerbate inflammation in the body. Conversely, an anti-inflammatory diet can help reduce the severity of psoriasis symptoms.

- **Immune System Function**: As an autoimmune disease, psoriasis is linked to immune system dysfunction. The immune system mistakenly targets healthy skin cells, leading to the characteristic red, scaly patches. Nutrition can influence the immune system's behavior. Consuming a diet rich in immune-boosting nutrients, such as vitamins C and D, can support a more balanced immune response and potentially reduce the autoimmune component of psoriasis.

- **Skin Health**: Nutrition directly impacts the health and integrity of the skin. Skin is the body's largest organ, and it requires essential nutrients to function optimally. Certain vitamins and minerals, like vitamin A, vitamin E, and zinc, are essential for skin health. A diet deficient in these nutrients can contribute to dry, itchy skin, which is a common complaint among those with psoriasis.

- **Gut-Immune Connection**: Research has unveiled the gut-immune-skin axis, emphasizing the interconnectedness of the gut, immune system, and skin health. The gut microbiome, which is influenced by diet, plays a significant role in regulating immune responses. An imbalanced gut microbiome can contribute to systemic inflammation, potentially worsening psoriasis symptoms. Probiotic-rich foods and a diet high in fiber can promote a healthier gut microbiome and indirectly benefit those with psoriasis.

- **Weight Management**: Obesity and excess body fat have been associated with an increased risk of psoriasis and more severe symptoms. A nutritious diet can help with weight management, which, in turn, can positively affect psoriasis. Losing excess weight through a balanced diet and regular physical activity can reduce inflammation and improve skin health.

2.2 Common Triggers and Aggravators

Psoriasis is a highly individualized condition, and what triggers or exacerbates symptoms can vary from person to person. However, there are some common dietary triggers and aggravators that individuals with psoriasis should be aware of:

- **High Sugar and Processed Foods**: Foods with a high sugar content and processed ingredients have been linked to increased inflammation. These foods can lead to spikes in blood sugar levels and may exacerbate psoriasis symptoms in some individuals.

- **Dairy Products**: Some people with psoriasis find that dairy products, particularly full-fat and high-lactose items, can trigger or worsen their symptoms. This may be due to the proteins and hormones in dairy that can impact inflammation and the immune system.

- **Red Meat**: Red meat, especially when it's high in saturated fats, can contribute to inflammation. It's advisable for individuals with psoriasis to limit their consumption of red meat and opt for leaner protein sources like poultry, fish, or plant-based proteins.

- **Alcohol**: Excessive alcohol consumption can trigger or worsen psoriasis in some individuals. Alcohol is known to dilate blood vessels, leading to an inflammatory response that can exacerbate skin symptoms.

- **Gluten**: While gluten sensitivity or celiac disease is not common in individuals with psoriasis, some may experience symptom improvement when avoiding gluten-containing foods. This suggests that a gluten-free diet may be beneficial for certain individuals.

- **Nightshade Vegetables**: Some people with psoriasis believe that nightshade vegetables like tomatoes, peppers, and eggplants may worsen their symptoms. While more research is needed to confirm this, it's worth considering these foods as potential triggers and avoiding them if they appear to exacerbate psoriasis.

The relationship between psoriasis and nutrition is a multifaceted one. Understanding how nutrition influences inflammation, the immune system, and skin health is critical for individuals with psoriasis. Identifying and avoiding common dietary triggers and aggravators can play a key role in managing and potentially reducing psoriasis symptoms. However, it's essential to remember that psoriasis is a highly individual condition, and what works for one person may not work for another. Personalized dietary choices should be made in consultation with a healthcare professional or registered dietitian to ensure they align with an individual's specific needs and circumstances.

2.3 The Connection Between Inflammation and Diet

Understanding the intricate relationship between inflammation and diet is essential when it comes to managing psoriasis, as this chronic skin condition is closely tied to an overactive inflammatory response within the body. In this section, we delve into the complex web of connections between diet and inflammation and how it pertains to psoriasis.

- **Chronic Inflammation**: Inflammation is a natural, protective response by the immune system that occurs when the body is under threat from injury, infection, or other stressors. It's characterized by redness, swelling, heat, and pain, which are signs that immune cells are actively working to repair and protect tissue. However, in conditions like psoriasis, inflammation becomes chronic and misdirected. Rather than defending against external threats, the immune system targets healthy skin cells, triggering a cascade of inflammation.

- **Pro-Inflammatory Foods**: Certain dietary choices can contribute to a pro-inflammatory state in the body. These choices often include foods high in sugar, refined carbohydrates, unhealthy fats, and additives. Such foods can prompt the release of pro-inflammatory substances in the body, exacerbating chronic inflammation. The frequent consumption of pro-inflammatory foods can make psoriasis symptoms more severe and resistant to treatment.

- **Anti-Inflammatory Foods**: Conversely, an anti-inflammatory diet is composed of foods that help reduce inflammation in the body. These foods are rich in antioxidants, omega-3 fatty acids, and essential vitamins and minerals. Consuming a diet rich in these anti-inflammatory nutrients can potentially dampen the inflammatory response in the body and, in turn, improve psoriasis symptoms.

- **Omega-3 Fatty Acids**: Omega-3 fatty acids are renowned for their anti-inflammatory properties. They can be found in fatty fish (e.g., salmon, mackerel), flaxseeds, chia seeds, and walnuts. The consumption of omega-3-rich foods or supplements can help balance the inflammatory response in the body, which may alleviate psoriasis symptoms for some individuals.

- **Antioxidants**: Antioxidant-rich foods, including a variety of fruits and vegetables, help counteract oxidative stress and reduce inflammation. Vitamins like vitamin C and E, as well as minerals like zinc, play critical roles in skin health and can be obtained from such foods.

- **Gut Health and Inflammation**: Emerging research has highlighted the connection between gut health and inflammation. The gut microbiome, the community of microorganisms in the digestive tract, plays a crucial role in regulating immune responses. An imbalanced or unhealthy gut microbiome can promote systemic inflammation, which may trigger or worsen psoriasis. A diet high in fiber and probiotic-rich foods supports a healthy gut microbiome, indirectly helping manage inflammation.

- **Hydration**: Proper hydration is often overlooked in discussions about diet and inflammation. Dehydrated skin is more prone to inflammation, redness, and itching. Staying well-hydrated by drinking sufficient water and consuming water-rich foods can help maintain skin moisture and reduce psoriasis-related discomfort.

The connection between inflammation and diet is a fundamental aspect of understanding psoriasis and its management. While dietary choices cannot cure psoriasis, they can significantly influence the severity and frequency of symptoms. By adopting an anti-inflammatory diet that includes foods rich in antioxidants, omega-3 fatty acids, and gut-healthy options, individuals with psoriasis can potentially reduce the chronic inflammation associated with the condition. Personalized dietary adjustments, combined with medical guidance and treatment, can contribute to better skin health and an improved overall quality of life for those living with psoriasis.

CHAPTER 3

The Psoriasis Diet Fundamentals

3.1 Balanced Nutrition for Psoriasis

Balanced nutrition is the cornerstone of an effective psoriasis diet. This section focuses on the importance of maintaining a balanced diet to support overall health and manage psoriasis symptoms. Here are some key points:

- **Variety and Moderation**: A balanced diet for psoriasis incorporates a variety of foods from different food groups, including fruits, vegetables, whole grains, lean proteins, and healthy fats. It's essential to enjoy a wide array of nutrients to support overall well-being.

- **Healthy Fats**: Opt for healthy fats, such as those found in avocados, nuts, seeds, and fatty fish like salmon. These fats can help reduce inflammation and maintain skin health.

- **Lean Proteins**: Protein is crucial for tissue repair and immune function. Choose lean sources of protein like poultry, fish, legumes, and tofu. Reducing red meat consumption can help manage inflammation.

- **Whole Grains**: Whole grains like quinoa, brown rice, and whole wheat provide essential nutrients and fiber, which promote gut health and may reduce inflammation.

- **Fruits and Vegetables**: The antioxidants and vitamins found in fruits and vegetables are essential for skin health. A colorful, plant-rich diet can provide a wide range of nutrients and help combat oxidative stress.

- **Portion Control**: Maintaining a healthy weight is essential for individuals with psoriasis, as excess body fat can exacerbate symptoms. Portion control is vital to avoid overeating and manage calorie intake.

3.2 Key Nutrients for Skin Health

The health of your skin, a critical concern for individuals with psoriasis, is closely tied to the consumption of specific nutrients. Here's a closer look at some of these key nutrients:

- **Vitamin A**: Vitamin A is essential for skin health and repair. It's found in foods like sweet potatoes, carrots, and dark leafy greens. Some individuals with psoriasis may benefit from vitamin A supplementation, but it's essential to consult a healthcare professional before doing so.

- **Vitamin E**: Vitamin E is an antioxidant that can help protect skin cells from damage. Foods like nuts, seeds, and

spinach are good sources.
Including these in your diet can
aid in maintaining healthy skin.

- **Vitamin C**: Vitamin C is vital
  for collagen production and
  plays a role in skin healing.
  Citrus fruits, strawberries, and
  bell peppers are rich sources of
  vitamin C.

- **Zinc**: Zinc is crucial for skin
  health and the immune system.
  It's found in foods like oysters,
  nuts, and whole grains.
  Adequate zinc intake can aid in
  skin repair and immunity.

- **Vitamin D**: Vitamin D plays a
  role in immune regulation, and
  some individuals with psoriasis
  have low vitamin D levels.
  Sunlight and fortified foods can
  be sources of vitamin D, but

supplementation may be necessary in consultation with a healthcare provider.

- **Selenium**: Selenium is an essential mineral that has antioxidant properties. It's found in foods like Brazil nuts, whole grains, and lean meats. Selenium may help reduce oxidative stress in the skin.

3.3 Portion Control and Meal Planning

Proper portion control and meal planning are essential components of a successful psoriasis diet. Here's a breakdown of these concepts:

- **Portion Control**: Monitoring portion sizes is critical for managing calorie intake and, subsequently, body weight. Overeating can lead to weight gain, which is a common trigger for psoriasis symptoms. Measuring portions and being mindful of portion sizes can help individuals maintain a healthy weight.

- **Balanced Meals**: Creating balanced meals that include a mix of lean proteins, complex carbohydrates, and healthy fats can provide sustained energy and support overall health. Balanced meals can help stabilize blood sugar levels and reduce the risk of inflammation triggered by blood sugar spikes.

- **Meal Planning**: Planning meals in advance ensures that individuals have access to healthy, psoriasis-friendly options. It can prevent impulsive choices that may not align with dietary goals. Meal planning also facilitates the incorporation of key nutrients essential for skin health.

- **Snacking**: For individuals with psoriasis, choosing healthy snacks between meals can help maintain energy levels and prevent overeating during main meals. Opt for nutritious snacks like fruits, yogurt, nuts, and vegetables with hummus.

The Psoriasis Diet Fundamentals emphasize the importance of balanced nutrition, key nutrients for skin health, and the significance of portion control and meal planning. By following these fundamentals, individuals with psoriasis can better manage their condition, reduce inflammation, and support overall well-being. However, it's essential to remember that dietary changes should be tailored to individual needs and consulted with a healthcare provider or registered dietitian to ensure they align with specific health goals and conditions.

CHAPTER 4

Foods to Include

4.1 Anti-Inflammatory Foods

Incorporating anti-inflammatory foods into your diet is a key strategy for managing psoriasis. These foods can help reduce the overall inflammatory load in your body, potentially leading to fewer flare-ups and milder symptoms. Here's a look at some anti-inflammatory foods:

- **Fruits**: Berries, cherries, and citrus fruits are rich in antioxidants and vitamin C, which can help reduce inflammation. Additionally, apples, particularly with the skin on, contain quercetin, a natural anti-inflammatory compound.

- **Vegetables**: Dark leafy greens, such as kale and spinach, are packed with vitamins and minerals that support skin health. Bell peppers, broccoli, and sweet potatoes provide antioxidants and vitamins A and C.

- **Fatty Fish**: Salmon, mackerel, sardines, and trout are excellent sources of omega-3 fatty acids, which have potent anti-inflammatory properties. These fatty acids can help mitigate inflammation and may alleviate psoriasis symptoms.

- **Nuts and Seeds**: Almonds, walnuts, and flaxseeds are rich in healthy fats and antioxidants. They are particularly high in omega-3 fatty acids and can be beneficial for reducing inflammation.

- **Turmeric**: This spice contains curcumin, a potent natural anti-inflammatory compound. Incorporating turmeric into your diet can have anti-inflammatory effects. Consider adding it to curries, soups, or smoothies.

- **Green Tea**: Green tea is known for its high levels of catechins, antioxidants that have anti-inflammatory properties. Drinking green tea regularly can contribute to a reduced inflammatory response.

- **Ginger**: Ginger is another spice with natural anti-inflammatory effects. It can be used in both cooking and tea to help reduce inflammation in the body.

- **Olive Oil**: Extra virgin olive oil is rich in monounsaturated fats and antioxidants, which can help lower inflammation. Use it as a cooking oil or drizzle it on salads.

- **Legumes**: Beans, lentils, and chickpeas are excellent sources of plant-based protein, fiber, and antioxidants. They support overall health and may help mitigate inflammation.

- **Probiotic-Rich Foods**: Fermented foods like yogurt, kefir, sauerkraut, and kimchi contain beneficial probiotics that support gut health. A healthy gut microbiome can indirectly reduce systemic inflammation.

4.2 Omega-3 Fatty Acids and Psoriasis

Omega-3 fatty acids are a standout among anti-inflammatory foods and are especially relevant for individuals with psoriasis. Here's why omega-3 fatty acids are beneficial:

- **Anti-Inflammatory Properties**: Omega-3 fatty acids, specifically eicosapentaenoic acid (EPA) and docosahexaenoic acid (DHA) found in fatty fish, have potent anti-inflammatory properties. These fatty acids can help reduce the production of inflammatory chemicals in the body.

- **Reduced Inflammatory Response**: Incorporating omega-3-rich foods or supplements into your diet can lead to a reduction in the severity and frequency of psoriasis symptoms. These fatty acids help modulate the immune response and inhibit the inflammatory cascade involved in psoriasis.

- **Improved Skin Health**: Omega-3 fatty acids contribute to healthier skin by maintaining its moisture and reducing dryness and itching, common concerns for individuals with psoriasis. These fatty acids also support the skin's barrier function, aiding in skin repair.

- **Food Sources**: Fatty fish like salmon, mackerel, sardines, and trout are the best dietary sources of omega-3 fatty acids. Plant-based sources include flaxseeds, chia seeds, walnuts, and hemp seeds. Fish oil supplements can also be considered under the guidance of a healthcare professional.

Including anti-inflammatory foods and omega-3 fatty acids in your diet is a proactive step in managing psoriasis. These foods can help reduce inflammation, mitigate psoriasis symptoms, and promote overall skin health. However, dietary changes should be made mindfully and in consultation with a healthcare provider or registered dietitian to ensure they align with your specific health needs and preferences.

4.3 Antioxidant-Rich Foods

Antioxidant-rich foods play a critical role in supporting skin health and managing psoriasis. These foods help combat oxidative stress, a common factor in inflammatory skin conditions like psoriasis. Here are some antioxidant-rich foods to include in your diet:

- **Berries**: Blueberries, strawberries, raspberries, and blackberries are packed with antioxidants such as anthocyanins and vitamin C. These compounds help protect

skin cells from damage caused
by free radicals.

- **Dark Leafy Greens**: Spinach,
  kale, and Swiss chard are
  excellent sources of
  antioxidants like lutein and
  zeaxanthin, which protect skin
  from oxidative stress and UV
  damage.

- **Colorful Vegetables**: Bell
  peppers, tomatoes, and carrots
  are rich in carotenoids like
  beta-carotene and lycopene.
  These antioxidants are known
  for their skin-protective
  properties.

- **Citrus Fruits**: Oranges,
  lemons, and grapefruits are
  high in vitamin C, a powerful
  antioxidant that promotes

collagen production and skin repair.

- **Nuts and Seeds**: Almonds, walnuts, and sunflower seeds are rich in vitamin E, which helps protect skin cells from oxidative damage.

- **Green Tea**: Green tea contains catechins, which are potent antioxidants that help maintain skin health and reduce inflammation.

- **Sweet Potatoes**: Rich in beta-carotene, sweet potatoes support skin cell turnover and repair.

- **Avocado**: Avocados provide vitamin E and healthy fats, both of which contribute to skin hydration and protection.

- **Broccoli**: Broccoli is a source of sulforaphane, an antioxidant with potential anti-inflammatory and skin-protective effects.

- **Pomegranates**: Pomegranates are rich in polyphenols, which have been associated with anti-inflammatory and antioxidant properties.

Including these antioxidant-rich foods in your diet can help reduce oxidative stress and support healthier skin. These foods are not only delicious but also offer numerous benefits for individuals with psoriasis.

4.4 Hydrating Your Skin through Diet

Maintaining skin hydration is crucial for individuals with psoriasis as dry, itchy skin is a common symptom. Your diet can play a significant role in skin hydration. Here's how you can use diet to keep your skin moisturized:

- **Water**: Staying well-hydrated by drinking an adequate amount of water is essential for maintaining skin moisture. Aim to consume at least eight glasses (about 2 liters) of water per day, more if you're physically active or in hot weather.

- **Water-Rich Foods**: Incorporate water-rich foods into your diet, such as cucumbers, watermelon, oranges, and strawberries. These foods not only contribute to hydration but also provide valuable antioxidants and nutrients for your skin.

- **Healthy Fats**: Omega-3 fatty acids found in fatty fish, flaxseeds, and walnuts can help maintain the skin's lipid barrier, preventing moisture loss and reducing dryness.

- **Avoid Dehydrating Foods**: Some foods can dehydrate the body, potentially exacerbating dry skin. Limit your consumption of caffeine and alcohol, as they can have a diuretic effect, leading to increased fluid loss.

- **Moisturizing Nutrients**:
  Include foods rich in vitamin E,
  such as almonds and sunflower
  seeds. Vitamin E can help
  maintain skin moisture and
  protect it from damage.

- **Probiotics**: A healthy gut
  microbiome can indirectly
  support skin hydration. Include
  probiotic-rich foods like yogurt
  and kefir to promote gut health.

Hydrating your skin through diet is a
valuable component of psoriasis
management. It can help alleviate the
discomfort of dry, itchy skin and
improve your overall skin health.
Combining dietary strategies with
topical moisturizers can be
particularly effective in keeping your
skin hydrated and comfortable.

Incorporating antioxidant-rich foods and hydrating your skin through diet is essential for individuals with psoriasis. These dietary strategies can help reduce oxidative stress, promote skin hydration, and contribute to healthier, more comfortable skin. As with any dietary changes, it's advisable to consult a healthcare provider or registered dietitian to tailor your diet to your specific health needs and preferences.

CHAPTER 5

Foods to Avoid

5.1 Common Psoriasis Triggers

For individuals with psoriasis, avoiding common triggers in their diet is crucial for managing symptoms and reducing the likelihood of flare-ups. Here are some common dietary triggers to be cautious of:

- **Processed Foods**: Highly processed and sugary foods can promote inflammation in the body. These include items like sugary snacks, fast food, and many packaged convenience foods. Excessive sugar intake may exacerbate psoriasis.

- **Alcohol**: Excessive alcohol consumption can dehydrate the body and lead to inflammation. Some individuals with psoriasis find that alcohol worsens their symptoms. Limiting or avoiding alcohol can be beneficial.

- **Red Meat**: Red meat, particularly when it's high in saturated fats, has been associated with inflammation. Some individuals may experience symptom improvement by reducing their consumption of red meat and choosing leaner protein sources.

- **Dairy Products**: Some people with psoriasis report that dairy products, especially full-fat and high-lactose items, trigger or worsen their symptoms. This could be due to the proteins and hormones in dairy that can impact inflammation and the immune system.

- **Gluten**: While psoriasis is not typically linked to gluten sensitivity or celiac disease, some individuals may experience symptom improvement when avoiding gluten-containing foods. It's worth considering a gluten-free diet if it seems to alleviate symptoms.

- **Nightshade Vegetables**: Some people with psoriasis believe that nightshade vegetables like tomatoes, peppers, and eggplants may exacerbate their symptoms. While more research is needed to confirm this, it's wise to consider these foods as potential triggers and avoid them if they appear to worsen psoriasis.

5.2 High-Inflammatory Foods

High-inflammatory foods are those that can exacerbate inflammation in the body, which is a significant concern for individuals with psoriasis. Steering clear of these foods can help manage psoriasis symptoms:

- **Trans Fats**: Trans fats are artificially created fats found in many fried and processed foods. They are known to promote inflammation and should be avoided.

- **Refined Carbohydrates**:
Foods made with refined
grains, such as white bread and
sugary cereals, can cause rapid
spikes in blood sugar levels,
potentially triggering
inflammation.

- **Sugary Snacks and
Beverages**: Excess sugar
intake, particularly from sugary
snacks, soda, and sweets, can
contribute to inflammation and
exacerbate psoriasis symptoms.

- **Excessive Omega-6 Fats**:
While omega-3 fatty acids
(found in fatty fish) are anti-
inflammatory, an imbalance
between omega-3 and omega-6
fats can promote inflammation.
Omega-6 fats are abundant in
many vegetable oils, so
reducing consumption of foods

cooked in these oils can help
balance the ratio.

- **Salt**: High-sodium diets can
  lead to water retention and
  exacerbate psoriasis-related
  swelling. Reducing salt intake
  by avoiding processed and salty
  foods is advisable.

5.3 The Role of Allergens

Allergens, particularly food allergens,
can play a role in the severity of
psoriasis symptoms for some
individuals. It's essential to be aware
of potential allergens and their
impact:

- **Food Allergies**: Some people
  with psoriasis may have
  sensitivities or allergies to
  specific foods. Common

allergens include nuts, shellfish, eggs, and dairy products. Identifying and avoiding allergenic foods can prevent allergic reactions that may worsen psoriasis.

- **Gluten Sensitivity**: While gluten sensitivity doesn't affect all individuals with psoriasis, some may find relief from their symptoms by adopting a gluten-free diet. If you suspect gluten sensitivity, consider working with a healthcare provider or dietitian for proper evaluation and guidance.

Being mindful of common psoriasis triggers, high-inflammatory foods, and potential allergens is essential for managing psoriasis effectively. While these dietary restrictions can help alleviate symptoms for many individuals, it's important to remember that psoriasis varies from person to person, and what works for one may not work for another. Personalized dietary choices should be made in consultation with a healthcare provider or registered dietitian to ensure they align with your specific needs and circumstances.

CHAPTER 6

Creating a Psoriasis-Friendly Meal Plan

6.1 Weekly Meal Planning

Weekly meal planning is a valuable strategy for individuals with psoriasis to ensure they follow a psoriasis-friendly diet consistently. Here's how to go about it:

- **Assess Your Goals**: Begin by assessing your dietary goals. Consider your specific psoriasis symptoms, overall health objectives, and any food restrictions or sensitivities. Determine whether you need to

lose weight, reduce
inflammation, or address other
health concerns alongside
psoriasis management.

- **Plan Balanced Meals**: Create
  balanced meals that include a
  mix of lean proteins, complex
  carbohydrates, and healthy fats.
  Ensure you include a variety of
  fruits and vegetables, whole
  grains, and omega-3-rich foods
  in your plan.

- **Include Anti-Inflammatory
  Foods**: Focus on incorporating
  anti-inflammatory foods like
  fatty fish, berries, dark leafy
  greens, nuts, seeds, and colorful
  vegetables into your meals.
  These foods can help reduce
  inflammation and support your
  skin health.

- **Avoid Triggers**: Be mindful of common psoriasis triggers and high-inflammatory foods. Plan meals that steer clear of processed foods, sugary snacks, alcohol, and other potential triggers. Opt for gluten-free and dairy-free alternatives if necessary.

- **Hydrating Options**: Include water-rich foods like cucumbers, watermelon, and citrus fruits to support skin hydration. Drinking an adequate amount of water is also essential for maintaining skin moisture.

- **Portion Control**: Ensure portion control to manage calorie intake and maintain a healthy weight. Monitoring portion sizes can help prevent overeating.

- **Variety**: Keep your meals interesting by varying your food choices. This not only prevents dietary boredom but also ensures you obtain a broad range of nutrients.

- **Meal Prepping**: Consider preparing meals in advance to make adhering to your psoriasis-friendly diet more convenient. Prepping meals and snacks for the week can help you avoid impulsive choices that may not align with your dietary goals.

- **Monitor Progress**: Keep a food diary to track your dietary choices and how they impact your psoriasis symptoms. This can provide valuable insights and help you refine your meal plan over time.

6.2 Sample Meal Plans

Here are two sample meal plans to provide a practical idea of how to create psoriasis-friendly meals:

Sample Meal Plan 1:

Breakfast:

- Scrambled eggs with spinach and tomatoes

- Whole-grain toast

- A side of berries

Lunch:

- Grilled chicken salad with mixed greens, bell peppers, and a vinaigrette dressing

- Quinoa or brown rice

Snack:

- Greek yogurt with honey and a handful of almonds

Dinner:

- Baked salmon with a lemon and dill sauce

- Steamed broccoli

- Sweet potato

Sample Meal Plan 2:

Breakfast:

- Oatmeal topped with fresh strawberries and a sprinkle of chia seeds

- A glass of freshly squeezed orange juice

Lunch:

- Lentil soup with a side of mixed greens and olive oil dressing

- A slice of whole-grain bread

Snack:

- Carrot sticks with hummus

Dinner:

- Grilled tofu with stir-fried vegetables (bell peppers, broccoli, snap peas) in a light ginger sauce

- Brown rice

These sample meal plans emphasize balanced, anti-inflammatory, and hydrating foods while avoiding common psoriasis triggers. Remember that these are just examples, and your meal plan should be personalized to your specific dietary needs and preferences. Consulting with a healthcare provider or registered dietitian can help you create a customized meal plan tailored to your psoriasis management goals.

6.3 Recipes and Cooking Tips

Certainly! Here are a few psoriasis-friendly recipes and cooking tips to help you create meals that support your psoriasis management:

Recipes:

1. Grilled Salmon with Lemon and Dill Sauce:

Ingredients:

- 4 salmon fillets
- Juice of 1 lemon

- 2 tablespoons of fresh dill, chopped

- 2 cloves of garlic, minced

- 2 tablespoons of olive oil

- Salt and pepper to taste

Instructions:

1. In a bowl, mix the lemon juice, chopped dill, minced garlic, and olive oil to create the sauce.

2. Season the salmon fillets with salt and pepper.

3. Preheat the grill to medium-high heat.

4. Place the salmon fillets on the grill and cook for about 4-5 minutes per side, or until the salmon is opaque and flakes easily.

5. Drizzle the lemon and dill sauce over the grilled salmon before serving.

2. Quinoa and Vegetable Salad:

Ingredients:

- 1 cup of quinoa

- 2 cups of water

- Mixed vegetables (e.g., bell peppers, cucumbers, cherry tomatoes)

- Fresh basil leaves, chopped

- Olive oil

- Balsamic vinegar

- Salt and pepper to taste

Instructions:

1. Rinse the quinoa under cold water. In a saucepan, combine

the quinoa and water, bring to a boil, then reduce the heat and simmer for about 15 minutes or until the quinoa is tender and the water is absorbed. Let it cool.

2. Dice the mixed vegetables and add them to the cooked and cooled quinoa.

3. Toss the salad with chopped fresh basil leaves.

4. Drizzle olive oil and balsamic vinegar over the salad and season with salt and pepper to taste. Mix well before serving.

Cooking Tips:

- **Use Healthy Cooking Methods**: Opt for healthy cooking methods like grilling, steaming, baking, and sautéing with olive oil instead of deep frying. These methods preserve the nutritional value of foods and reduce the consumption of unhealthy fats.

- **Season with Herbs and Spices**: Instead of salt or excessive seasoning, use herbs and spices like turmeric, ginger, garlic, and rosemary to add flavor to your dishes. Many herbs and spices have anti-inflammatory properties.

- **Substitute Dairy**: If you're sensitive to dairy or want to reduce dairy consumption, try dairy-free alternatives like almond milk, coconut yogurt, or cashew-based cheese in your recipes.

- **Explore Whole Grains**: Replace refined grains with whole grains like quinoa, brown rice, and whole wheat pasta. These grains provide more fiber and essential nutrients.

- **Incorporate Omega-3 Foods**: Include fatty fish like salmon, mackerel, and sardines in your diet regularly to benefit from their omega-3 fatty acids. If you prefer plant-based sources, try flaxseeds, chia seeds, and walnuts.

- **Stay Hydrated**: Alongside meals, remember to maintain proper hydration. Drinking sufficient water is essential for skin health. You can also enjoy hydrating foods like water-rich fruits and vegetables.

- **Limit Alcohol**: If you consume alcohol, do so in moderation. Overindulgence in alcohol can lead to inflammation and may exacerbate psoriasis symptoms.

By following these recipes and cooking tips, you can create delicious and psoriasis-friendly meals that promote skin health and reduce inflammation. Remember to personalize your meals to align with your specific dietary needs and consult with a healthcare provider or registered dietitian for further guidance and support in managing your psoriasis through diet.

CHAPTER 7

Lifestyle and Psoriasis Management

7.1 Stress Management

Stress management is a vital component of psoriasis management because stress can trigger or exacerbate psoriasis symptoms. Here are strategies for effectively managing stress:

- **Meditation and Mindfulness**: Practices like meditation and mindfulness can help reduce stress and promote relaxation. These techniques focus on being present in the moment and can reduce anxiety and tension.

- **Yoga**: Yoga combines physical postures, breathing exercises, and meditation. It is known to reduce stress and promote flexibility and balance.

- **Breathing Exercises**: Simple deep breathing exercises can be done anywhere and anytime to help you relax and alleviate stress.

- **Physical Activity**: Regular physical activity, such as walking, jogging, or swimming, releases endorphins, which are natural mood boosters. Exercise can help reduce stress and improve overall well-being.

- **Counseling or Therapy**: If stress is a significant factor in your life, consider seeking support from a therapist or counselor who can help you address the underlying causes of stress and develop effective coping strategies.

- **Time Management**: Organizing your time and setting priorities can reduce stress related to work and daily responsibilities.

- **Support Network**: Share your feelings and experiences with friends and family who can provide emotional support. Joining a psoriasis support group can also be valuable.

7.2 Exercise and Psoriasis

Regular exercise is a positive lifestyle choice for individuals with psoriasis. Here's how it can benefit your psoriasis management:

- **Stress Reduction**: As mentioned earlier, exercise can help reduce stress, which is a common trigger for psoriasis flare-ups. The release of endorphins during exercise promotes relaxation.

- **Weight Management**: Maintaining a healthy weight is important for individuals with psoriasis, as excess body fat can exacerbate symptoms. Exercise supports weight management and overall health.

- **Improved Circulation**: Exercise promotes better circulation, which can help the body deliver nutrients and oxygen to skin cells, potentially aiding in skin repair.

- **Anti-Inflammatory Effects**: Regular physical activity can have anti-inflammatory effects. It helps balance the immune system and reduce systemic inflammation.

- **Increased Energy**: Exercise can boost your energy levels, which can be beneficial for those dealing with psoriasis-related fatigue.

- **Enhanced Mental Health**: The psychological benefits of exercise include improved mood and a sense of well-

being, which can be particularly
valuable for individuals
managing chronic conditions
like psoriasis.

It's essential to choose exercise that
you enjoy, as this increases the
likelihood that you will stick with it.
Whether it's walking, jogging,
swimming, yoga, or any other
physical activity, consistency is key.

7.3 Sleep and Skin Health

Adequate sleep is crucial for overall
health and can significantly impact
psoriasis management. Here's how to
ensure better sleep and its benefits for
skin health:

- **Establish a Sleep Routine**: Go
  to bed and wake up at the same
  time each day, even on

weekends. A regular sleep schedule helps regulate your body's internal clock.

- **Create a Relaxing Bedtime Routine**: Engage in calming activities before bedtime, such as reading, taking a warm bath, or practicing relaxation exercises. Avoid stimulating activities like working on a computer or watching intense TV shows.

- **Maintain a Comfortable Sleep Environment**: Ensure your sleep environment is conducive to rest. This includes a comfortable mattress, appropriate room temperature, and minimal light and noise.

- **Limit Screen Time**: Exposure to the blue light emitted by screens can disrupt your sleep. Try to avoid screens (phones, tablets, computers, and TV) at least an hour before bedtime.

- **Monitor Your Diet**: Avoid heavy, large meals within a few hours of bedtime. Limit caffeine and alcohol intake in the evening, as they can interfere with sleep.

- **Manage Stress**: Effective stress management techniques, as discussed earlier, can significantly improve your sleep quality.

The benefits of good sleep include improved immune function, reduced inflammation, and enhanced skin health. A good night's sleep can help manage psoriasis symptoms and promote overall well-being.

lifestyle choices, such as stress management, regular exercise, and maintaining healthy sleep patterns, play an essential role in psoriasis management. By incorporating these practices into your daily life, you can reduce the likelihood of psoriasis flare-ups and improve your overall quality of life.

CHAPTER 8

Supplements and Psoriasis

8.1 Vitamins and Minerals

Certain vitamins and minerals can be beneficial for individuals with psoriasis. However, it's important to consult with a healthcare provider before adding supplements to your diet to ensure they align with your specific needs and health goals. Here are some vitamins and minerals to consider:

- **Vitamin D**: Some individuals with psoriasis have low vitamin D levels. Vitamin D

supplements may be prescribed
by a healthcare provider to
address deficiency. Adequate
vitamin D can help modulate
the immune response and
reduce inflammation.

- **Omega-3 Fatty Acids**: Omega-3 supplements, typically sourced from fish oil, can be used to increase the intake of these anti-inflammatory fatty acids. Omega-3s can help reduce inflammation and alleviate psoriasis symptoms. Consult with your healthcare provider for the appropriate dosage.

- **Vitamin A**: Vitamin A is essential for skin health and repair. However, excessive vitamin A supplementation can be harmful, so it should be used under the guidance of a healthcare provider.

- **Zinc**: Zinc is crucial for skin health and the immune system. Some individuals with psoriasis may benefit from zinc supplementation, but it should be done under the supervision of a healthcare provider.

- **Selenium**: Selenium is an essential mineral with antioxidant properties. Adequate selenium intake can help reduce oxidative stress in the skin. Consult your healthcare provider for personalized advice.

- **Vitamin E**: Vitamin E is an antioxidant that can protect skin cells from damage. It can be obtained from dietary sources, but in some cases, supplementation may be recommended.

- **B Vitamins**: B vitamins, particularly vitamin B12 and folate, play a role in skin health and may be considered for supplementation if there is a deficiency.

8.2 Herbal Supplements

Several herbal supplements have been studied for their potential benefits in managing psoriasis. However, it's essential to consult with a healthcare provider before using herbal supplements, as they may interact with medications or have side effects. Here are some herbal supplements to consider:

- **Turmeric**: Curcumin, the active compound in turmeric, has anti-inflammatory properties and may help reduce psoriasis symptoms. Turmeric supplements are available, but their efficacy can vary. Consult with your healthcare provider for guidance.

- **Aloe Vera**: Aloe vera gel can be applied topically to soothe skin irritation caused by psoriasis. There are also aloe vera supplements available, but their effectiveness for internal use is less clear.

- **Milk Thistle**: Milk thistle supplements are believed to have potential liver-protective effects, which can be relevant for individuals with psoriasis. The liver plays a role in detoxification, and liver function may impact psoriasis. Consult your healthcare provider for recommendations.

- **Oregon Grape**: Oregon grape extract is sometimes used as a topical treatment for psoriasis. Some individuals use it internally, but it should be discussed with a healthcare provider.

- **Probiotics**: Probiotic supplements can support gut health, which indirectly affects skin health. An imbalanced gut microbiome can contribute to inflammation. Probiotics may be beneficial when recommended by a healthcare provider.

8.3 Consultation with a Healthcare Provider

Before taking any supplements for psoriasis, it's crucial to consult with a healthcare provider, preferably a dermatologist or a registered dietitian who specializes in psoriasis management. They can help you make informed decisions based on your individual health status, potential deficiencies, and the specific goals you want to achieve.

Your healthcare provider can:

- Assess your current health and nutritional status.

- Recommend appropriate supplements if deficiencies are identified.

- Provide guidance on dosage and duration.

- Ensure that supplements do not interact with any medications you may be taking.

- Monitor your progress and adjust recommendations as needed.

while vitamins, minerals, and herbal supplements may have potential benefits for individuals with psoriasis, they should be used judiciously and under the guidance of a healthcare provider. Always prioritize a balanced diet as the primary source of nutrients, and consider supplementation when it aligns with your specific health needs and is recommended by a qualified professional.

CHAPTER 9

Personalizing Your Psoriasis Diet

9.1 Keeping a Food Diary

Keeping a food diary is a valuable tool for personalizing your psoriasis diet. Here's how to do it effectively:

- **Document Your Meals**: Record everything you eat and drink, including portion sizes and preparation methods. Be as detailed as possible.

- **Include Timing**: Note the times at which you consume your meals and snacks. This can help identify any patterns in your diet and psoriasis symptoms.

- **Monitor Symptoms**: In addition to tracking your dietary intake, record your psoriasis symptoms and their severity. Common symptoms to track include redness, itching, inflammation, and flare-ups.

- **Assess Environmental Factors**: Document external factors like weather conditions, stress levels, and sleep patterns, as these can also affect psoriasis symptoms.

- **Use a Digital or Physical Diary**: You can keep a food diary using a dedicated app, a spreadsheet, or a physical notebook. Choose a method that's convenient for you.

- **Be Consistent**: Make an effort to record your meals consistently for at least a few weeks. Consistency is key to identifying patterns.

9.2 Tracking Psoriasis Symptoms

Tracking your psoriasis symptoms can help you understand how your diet affects your condition. Here's how to effectively monitor your symptoms:

- **Severity**: Rate the severity of your symptoms on a scale from 1 to 10, with 1 being the mildest and 10 being the most severe.

- **Location**: Note the specific areas on your body where

psoriasis symptoms are present. Some individuals may experience symptoms on their elbows, knees, scalp, or other areas.

- **Frequency**: Record how often you experience flare-ups or changes in your psoriasis symptoms.

- **Duration**: Document how long each episode of psoriasis lasts. This can help you identify any potential triggers.

- **Changes Over Time**: Observe if your symptoms change over time, and take note of any patterns that emerge.

9.3 Adjusting Your Diet as Needed

Once you've maintained a food diary and tracked your psoriasis symptoms, you can personalize your diet based on your observations. Here's how to make informed dietary adjustments:

- **Identify Triggers**: Look for patterns in your food diary that may be linked to psoriasis flare-ups or increased symptoms. Common triggers can include specific foods or food groups.

- **Experiment with Elimination**: Based on your identified triggers, consider eliminating or reducing those foods from your diet. This should be done gradually and under the

guidance of a healthcare
provider or dietitian.

- **Introduce Potential Beneficial Foods**: Incorporate anti-inflammatory and skin-friendly foods into your diet. Experiment with including more fruits, vegetables, fatty fish, and whole grains.

- **Consult a Healthcare Provider or Dietitian**: To make significant dietary changes, consult with a healthcare provider or a registered dietitian who specializes in psoriasis management. They can provide personalized recommendations and ensure that your dietary changes align with your overall health goals.

- **Monitor Progress**: Continue tracking your psoriasis symptoms and dietary changes. Assess whether the adjustments you've made have a positive or negative impact on your condition.

- **Be Patient**: It may take time to see noticeable improvements, and individual responses to dietary changes can vary. Consistency and patience are essential.

- **Consider All Aspects of Health**: Remember that psoriasis is influenced by various factors, including genetics, stress, and environmental factors. Your diet is just one aspect of your psoriasis management plan.

personalizing your psoriasis diet involves keeping a food diary, tracking psoriasis symptoms, and making informed dietary adjustments based on your observations. It's a gradual and ongoing process that should be done in collaboration with a healthcare provider or registered dietitian to ensure that your dietary choices align with your specific needs and goals.